I0096733

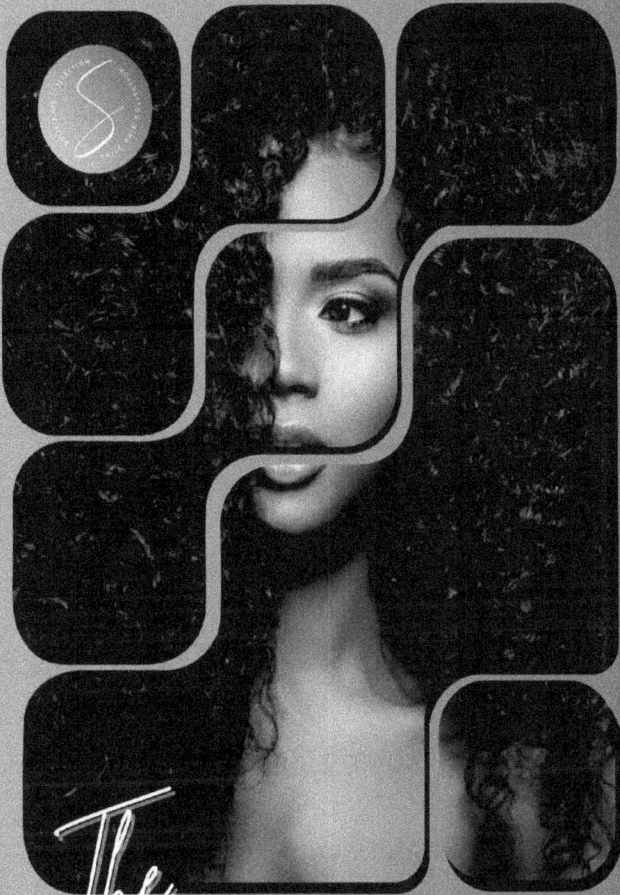

The
Ultimate Tape In Hair Guide

HOW TO INSTALL, MAINTAIN, AND REMOVE WITH EASE

Shawnta Auston

THE ULTIMATE
TAPE IN HAIR GUIDE

Copyright © 2023
Sasha's Savvy Solutions
All Rights Reserved

ISBN 979-8-9903694-0-5

Scan to learn more about
Sajje Hair Collection.
Check out our tutorials, videos, and
other info about our community.

www.sajjecollection.com

TABLE OF CONTENTS

TABLE OF CONTENTS

INTRODUCTION

As a hair extensions connoisseur, with over 15 years of experience and a successful hair extensions line under my belt, I am delighted to share with you the wonders of Tape In Hair Extensions, or as they are commonly referred to, "Tape Ins". These extensions have become incredibly popular and it's easy to see why. Not only are they a breeze to install, but they also provide a seamless, natural look that is perfect for those seeking to add volume and length to their hair.

Let's dive in..... What exactly are Tape In Hair Extensions? Simply put, they are hair extensions that use a strong, medical-grade adhesive tape to attach the extension to the natural hair. Unlike other extension methods, tape in extensions can be installed quickly, taking as little as an hour, sometimes a bit longer. This makes them a popular choice for individuals who are seeking a quick and easy solution.

What's more, tape in extensions are a versatile option that can be styled just like natural hair. The installation process is also pain-free, which is music to the ears of those who may have experienced discomfort with other extension methods.

Tape in extensions are a great choice for individuals looking to add length and volume to their hair without committing to more permanent options. Plus, the fact that they can be styled to match the natural hair makes them an attractive option. If you're in the market for hair extensions, give Tape In Hair Extensions a try - you won't be disappointed. And, if you want to ensure you're using the highest quality hair extensions available, I highly recommend the SHC Premium Tape In Hair Extensions by Sajje Hair Collection

Chapter 1

Introduction
to
Tape In Hair Extensions

Welcome! In this Chapter, we will introduce you to this popular hair extension method and explore its benefits.

Hair extensions have been a favorite beauty accessory for many years, offering a quick and easy way to change your look, add volume, length, or color to the natural hair. Tape in hair extensions, in particular, have been gaining popularity since their introduction in 2010 as a more natural, low-damage alternative to other extension methods.

One of the main reasons why tape in extensions have become so popular is because of their ease of installation and minimal damage to natural hair. Unlike other methods, such as bonding or weaving, tape in extensions do not require heat, chemicals or sewing, reducing the risk of damage. Additionally, they are made of 100% human hair, which allows for seamless blending with natural hair, creating a more natural-looking hairstyle.

Moreover, tape in extensions offer versatility in styling options, as they can be washed, blow-dried, and styled just like natural hair. They are also easy to install and remove, making them a popular choice for DIY enthusiasts.

In the following chapters of this guide, we will delve deeper into the installation and removal process of tape in extensions, as well as provide tips and tricks for maintenance and care.

Stay tuned

Chapter 2

Assessing
Tape In Hair Extension
Quality

Selecting high-quality tape in hair extensions is essential to achieve the desired look and durability. Therefore, it is important to know how to assess them properly to make an informed decision.

Factors to Consider When Selecting Tape In Hair Extensions

First, the quality of the hair used is one of the most critical factors to consider when selecting tape in hair extensions. High-quality extensions are made with 100% Remy human hair, which means that the hair cuticles are aligned in the same direction, resulting in a natural-looking, shiny, and soft texture.

Additionally, the tape used to attach the extensions should be strong, durable, and easy to remove without damaging the natural hair. It should also be hypoallergenic and safe for sensitive skin. The length and thickness of the extensions should closely match the natural hair in order to achieve a seamless and natural look, and the installation process should be easy and straightforward.

How to Identify High-Quality Tape In Hair Extensions

To identify high-quality tape in hair extensions, you can start by running your fingers through the hair to test its texture and quality. The hair should have a natural-looking texture that matches the natural hair, and the cuticles should be intact and aligned in the same direction. High-quality tape in hair extensions should not shed excessively and should last for several weeks without requiring frequent maintenance or replacement. They should also withstand heat styling and other styling products without becoming damaged or frizzy.

Common Signs of Low-Quality Tape In Hair Extensions

Low-quality tape in hair extensions may have a short lifespan, lasting only a few weeks or days before requiring replacement. They may also have an unnatural appearance, such as a shiny or synthetic texture that does not blend well with the natural hair.

SHC Premium Tape In Hair Extensions by Sajje Hair Collection

If you are looking for high-quality tape in hair extensions, I highly recommend the SHC Premium Tape In Hair Extensions by Sajje Hair Collection. These extensions are made from 100% Remy human hair, ensuring their highest quality. They are designed to last for up to 12 months with proper care and maintenance, making them a great investment for anyone who wants to add length and volume to their hair without sacrificing quality. The tapes used to secure the extensions are strong and durable, making them easy to apply and remove without causing any damage to the natural hair. The SHC Premium Tape In Hair Extensions come in a wide range of colors and lengths, making it easy to find the perfect match for the hair.

Tips for Selecting the Right Tape In Hair Extensions

When selecting tape in hair extensions, it is essential to choose high-quality extensions that blend well with the natural hair and last longer. Additionally, select tape in hair extensions that closely match the natural hair texture and color for a seamless and natural look. With these tips, you are one step closer to achieving the desired look and durability with tape in hair extensions.

Chapter 3

Preparing For
Tape In Hair Extensions

As you prepare for the installation of tape in hair extensions, it is vital to take the necessary steps to ensure a successful outcome. In order to do so, you must assess the health of the hair and scalp, choose the right extensions, and gather the proper tools for installation and removal.

Before installing tape in hair extensions, it's essential to evaluate the condition of the hair and scalp. This will help you avoid potential damage to the natural hair and ensure that the tape in extensions blend seamlessly. Take into account factors such as hair texture and color, and examine the scalp for any signs of irritation, inflammation, or infection. If you notice any issues, it's best to wait until the scalp is healthy before installing the extensions.

Next, gather the tools you'll need for the installation and removal process. A tail comb, sectioning clips, high-quality tape in hair extensions that match the hair color and texture, tape tabs, scissors, and solvent solution are all essential items. These tools will allow you to create sections in the hair, attach the extensions, and remove them without causing damage to the natural hair.

As we mentioned previously, consider using SHC Premium Tape In Hair Extensions by Sajje Hair Collection. These tape in hair extensions are made with high-quality materials that will blend seamlessly with the natural hair and have proven to be a fan fave. Additionally, Sajje Hair Collection offers an all⬛natural solvent solution that will minimize damage to the natural hair while moisturizing and conditioning it at the same time

By using the right tools and products, you can achieve a flawless tape in hair extension installation that will enhance your natural beauty.

Chapter 4

The Installation Process

Before starting the installation process, it's important to have all the necessary tools such as tape in hair extensions, tail comb, sectioning clips, Velcro grippers, tape in adhesive remover, rubbing alcohol, and tape in hair extension pliers. Also, ensure that the hair is freshly washed with no additional conditioner, serum, oil, or hair product added to hair or scalp prior to installation. This helps the tape adhesive to stick properly, making the tape in hair extension more secure and preventing it from slipping out.

Step 1:
Divide the hair into sections. Create a vertical part on each side of the head just behind each ear and a horizontal part approximately an inch above the nape of the neck. Braid or clip sectioned areas away from the hair where tape ins will be installed.

Step 2:
Prep the hair. Use a tail comb to create a horizontal part in the hair above the nape of the neck. Use a sectioning clip to hold the top part of the hair away from the bottom section. Ensure that the hair is clean and free of any dirt, debris, oil, or hair products. This step ensures that the tape will stick to the hair correctly.

Step 3:
Secure the hair. Prior to applying each tape in, it's important to use the necessary clips and Velcro grippers to secure and contain any loose or flyaway hair strands away from the section where the tape in is being installed. This will prevent any discomfort or potential hair loss if caught in between the tape and pulled the wrong way.

Step 4:
Apply the tape in hair extension. It's essential to ensure that the width for each section of natural hair is slightly less than the width of the tape in hair extension. This allows you to secure the tape tabs towards each end. Also, the natural hair being secured between the two tape tabs should not be too thick, as it will prevent the tape tabs from fully securing to each other. We recommend just enough hair to be able to secure to the natural hair while still having enough tape visibility so that the tabs can connect, attach to the opposite side, and remain secure for the install.

Remove the protective covering from one side of the tape. Be sure to barely touch the end of the tape tab upon removal of the covering, so as not to compromise the adhesive. Carefully place the tape onto the roots of the hair. Each tab should be applied leaving a small space, roughly the depth of a tail comb or about 1/8 of an inch. This will alleviate irritation to the scalp and prevent damage to the hair, which can result from the tape tabs being installed too closely to the scalp. Be sure to press it firmly, ideally with tape in pliers, so it adheres correctly. Remove the protective covering from the other tape in, place the tape in hair extension over the previously installed tape in adhesive, and press it down firmly. This creates what is called a sandwich.

Step 5:
Repeat the process. Continue applying tape in hair extensions to each section. Each tape in extension on a horizontal row should have just enough space to fit the side of your pinky finger between the next tape in. Move any flyaway hairs that are not intended for the section that you are working on. Continue working your way up the head and to each side section until you have the desired volume and length. For each side section, leave about an inch wide section of hair from the front hairline/face area, so that you will be able to cover the side tape ins as needed.

Pro Tip:
It's important to ensure that you are leaving enough hair out when installing around the nape and sides. Take the tail comb and lay the tail along the scalp, close to the root of the natural hair. Pull the "leave out" hair over the tail comb as if to cover it. If you are unable to see the tail comb through thenatural hair, it is safe to say that you've allowed enough "leave out" to cover the tape ins and prevent them from being seen while styling the hair.

Tips for Achieving a Natural Look with Tape In Hair Extensions

To achieve a natural look with tape in hair extensions, don't forget to follow these tips:

1. Match the color of the hair extensions to the natural hair color.
This ensures that the hair extensions blend seamlessly with the natural hair.

2. Cut the hair extensions to blend with the natural hair.
Once the hair extensions are installed, they may be longer than the natural hair. To ensure a natural look, cut and shape the hair extensions to blend with the natural hair length.

3. Avoid using too many hair extensions.
Using too many hair extensions may make the hair look fake and unnatural. Use only the number of hair extensions necessary to achieve your desired volume and length.

4. Use high-quality tape in hair extensions.
High-quality hair extensions are less likely to tangle or shed, and they will look more natural.

5. Don't forget to maintain the hair extensions. Proper maintenance will help the hair extensions last longer and look better. Avoid using heat styling tools too frequently, and be gentle when brushing and detangling the hair.

Troubleshooting Common Issues During Installation

Even with proper installation, you may encounter some common issues. Here are some tips for troubleshooting these issues:

1. Tape in hair extensions slipping out:
This can happen if the adhesive isn't strong enough. Make sure to use high-quality tape in hair extensions and follow the installation instructions carefully. You may also need to avoid using hair products on the hair or scalp prior to installation.

2. Tape in hair extensions feeling uncomfortable:
This can happen if the tape tabs are too close to the scalp or if too much hair is secured between the two tape tabs. Make sure to leave a small space between each tape tab and avoid securing too much hair between the tabs

3. Tape in hair extensions are visible:
This can happen if the hair extensions aren't cut or blended properly. Make sure to cut and shape the hair extensions to blend with the natural hair and follow the pro tip referenced previously, for leaving enough hair out around the nape and sides. Installing tape in hair extensions can be a great way to add length and volume to the hair. It is important to have all the necessary tools and to properly prep the hair before starting the installation process. Taking your time and being careful when applying the extensions will ensure that they stay securely in place and blend seamlessly with the natural hair. By following the tips for achieving a natural look, you can have beautiful, long, and full hair that looks and feels completely natural.

Chapter 5

Post Installation Care

It is extremely important to take great care of the hair and extensions after installation. When making the investment in hair extensions, you want to do what it takes to keep the extensions looking their best for as long as possible, while most importantly, caring for the natural hair.

In this chapter, we will share everything you need to know about post-installation care for the tape in extensions. From recommended products to styling tips and maintenance techniques, we've got you covered!

First things first, let's talk about taking care of the hair and extensions during the first few days after installation. The scalp may be sensitive, and the adhesive used to secure the extensions may still be setting, so it's crucial to take extra care during this time. Avoid washing the hair or getting it wet for at least 48 hours after installation to allow the adhesive to set fully.

Once the first 48 hours have passed, you can start washing the hair and extensions as normal. However, it's essential to use a sulfate-free shampoo and conditioner to avoid drying out the extensions or causing slippage. Be gentle when washing, massaging the shampoo into the scalp and hair, avoiding pulling or tugging on the extensions. Rinse thoroughly and apply conditioner, focusing on the mid-lengths and ends of the hair. Rinse again and gently squeeze out excess water.

When drying the hair, it's best to avoid using a hairdryer on high heat, as this can cause impact the integrity of the extensions, as well as your natural hair. Instead, gently squeeze out any excess water and wrap the hair in a microfiber towel or t-shirt to absorb the moisture. Once most of the moisture is absorbed, let the hair air-dry or use a hair dryer on a medium or low setting.

Now let's talk about recommended products for maintenance and styling. Using the right products can make a huge difference in the longevity and appearance of the tape in extensions. Here are some of our top picks:

1. Extension-Safe Shampoo and Conditioner:
Look for products specifically labeled as "extension safe" or "sulfate-free" to keep the extensions looking their best.

2. Leave-In Conditioner or Detangler:

A good leave-in conditioner can help detangle the hair and extensions and protect them from heat damage when styling. We like Aunt Jackie's "Knot On My Watch" Instant Detangling Therapy.

3. Heat Protectant:

To avoid damaging the extensions when using hot styling tools, such as curling irons or straighteners, use a heat protectant spray or serum. We recommend ORS Heat Protectant.

4. Hair Oil:

Applying a small amount of hair oil to the mid-lengths and ends of the hair can help keep the extensions soft, shiny, and tangle-free.

And here are some tips for extending the lifespan of the tape in hair extensions.

1. Avoid Sleeping with Wet Hair:

Sleeping with wet hair can cause tangles and knots, which can damage the extensions over time. Make sure to dry the hair thoroughly before going to bed, and consider putting it up in a loose braid or ponytail to prevent tangling or wrapping in a satin scarf or bonnet.

2. Don't Overwash The Hair:

Overwashing can strip the hair and extensions of natural oils, causing them to become dry and brittle. Try to wash the hair no more than twice a week, and use dry shampoo in between washes if needed.

3. Be Gentle When Brushing:

Use a soft-bristled brush or a wide-tooth comb to gently brush the hair and extensions, starting at the ends and working your way up.

4. Avoid Chemical Treatments:
Chemical treatments such as coloring, perming, or relaxing can weaken the adhesive used to attach the extensions, causing them to loosen or fall out.

5. Avoid Chlorine and Saltwater:
Chlorine and saltwater can cause damage to the extensions and dry out the natural hair. It's best to avoid swimming in pools or oceans while wearing tape in hair extensions. If you do go for a swim, be sure to wear a swim cap to protect the extensions and wash them thoroughly with sulfate-free shampoo and conditioner as soon as possible after swimming.

6. Protect The Extensions from Sun Damage:
Just like your natural hair, tape in hair extensions can also be damaged by prolonged exposure to the sun's harmful UV rays. If you plan to spend time outdoors, protect the extensions by wearing a hat or a scarf. You can also apply a leave-in conditioner with UV protection to help keep the extensions safe from the sun.

7. Use Oil-Based Products Sparingly:
While hair oil can help keep the extensions soft and shiny, it's important not to overdo it. Using too much oil-based products can weigh down the extensions and make them look greasy or clumpy. Use only a small amount of oil and apply it to the mid-lengths and ends of the hair.

8. Store The Extensions Properly:
When not in use, it's essential to store the tape in extensions properly to prevent damage and maintain their shape. Make sure to brush out any tangles or knots and store them in a clean, dry place, away from direct sunlight and heat sources. Sajje Hair Collection offers a handy storage bag, perfect for storing hair extensions when not in use.

Remember, proper post-installation care is essential for maintaining the quality and longevity of the tape in hair extensions. We know how important it is to take care of the hair and extensions to keep them looking their best and protect your investment. With a little extra care and attention, you can enjoy beautiful, natural-looking hair for weeks or even months. Don't forget to schedule regular maintenance appointments with a stylist or for your clients, to keep the extensions looking their best and to prevent damage to the natural hair.

Chapter 6

Preparing for Tape In Hair Extension Removal

Here we will guide you through the intricate process of tape in hair extension removal. It is of paramount importance to have a proper understanding of when and how to remove tape in hair extensions, in order to prevent damage to the natural hair and ensure a successful removal process.

To begin with, let us delve into the crucial process of assessing when the tape in hair extensions need to be removed. The lifespan of tape in hair extensions is influenced by various factors such as the quality of the extensions, the type of tape used, and how well they are maintained. On average, tape in hair extensions can last up to 6-8 weeks before they need to be removed and reinstalled. However, it is important to keep a watchful eye out for the following signs, which can indicate that it is time to remove the tape in hair extensions:

1. Slipping:
If you observe that the extensions are starting to slip or come loose, it is an indication that it's time to remove them. This can occur when the tape loses its adhesive properties or when the extensions have grown out too much.

2. Tangling:
If the extensions are becoming increasingly tangled, it can be a sign that they need to be removed. Tangled extensions can be a bane for the natural hair and can be difficult to brush out. Moreover, when the natural hair is prone to tangling, it can exacerbate the situation further.

3. Discomfort:
If you start to experience discomfort or pain while wearing the tape in hair extensions, it's time to remove them. This can be a sign that the extensions are pulling on the natural hair or scalp, which can cause damage and discomfort.

Next, let's take a look at the tools that are needed for the removal of tape in hair extensions. Before removing the tape in hair extensions, it is essential to have a few essential tools at hand, which include:

1. Tape in Hair Extension Remover:
This is a specially formulated solution designed to break down the adhesive in the tape, making it easier to remove the extensions. Sajje Hair Collection Tape In Hair Extension Remover is an excellent all-natural option that not only breaks down the adhesive but also moisturizes the natural hair.

2. Fine-tooth Comb or Soft Brush:
A fine-tooth comb or soft brush will help you gently comb out any tangles in the natural hair before and after removal.

3. Sectioning Clips:
Sectioning clips will help you separate the hair into manageable sections during the removal process.

Finally, let's delve into the tips for preparing the hair and scalp for tape in hair extension removal. Proper preparation of the hair and scalp can make the process go more smoothly and minimize damage to the natural hair. Here are a few tips to help you prepare:

1. Brush Hair Thoroughly:
Before starting the removal process, make sure to brush the hair thoroughly to remove any tangles or knots.

2. Assess Natural Hair When Removing:
When removing the extensions, use caution to avoid pulling or tugging on the natural hair. Gently work the remover solution into the tape and use a fine-tooth comb to separate the tape from the natural hair.

By following these steps and tips, you can successfully prepare for tape in hair extension removal and minimize any potential damage to the natural hair

Chapter 7

Tape In Hair Extension Removal Process

We understand and appreciate the importance of following the right process when it comes to removing tape in hair extensions. Not only can this help preserve the natural hair, but it can also ensure that the tape in hair extensions are in good condition for future use

To get started with the tape in hair extension removal process, it's important to gather all the necessary tools. Make sure you have a tail comb, Sajje Hair Collection Tape In Hair Extension Remover solution, a soft-bristled brush or make-up brush, and a spray bottle filled with alcohol on hand before starting.

Once you have all the necessary tools, it's time to section the hair into several sections and secure them with hair ties or clips. This will make it easier to work on each section individually and prevent tangling while removing each row of tape in hair.

Next, gently apply the Sajje Hair Collection Tape In Hair Extension Remover solution between the tape tabs of the extensions, using the narrow squirt tip, making sure to saturate the tape bond completely. Wait for the solution to soak in and loosen the adhesive. It usually takes between 5 to 10 minutes for the adhesive remover to break down the glue.

Once the bond has loosened, gently separate the tape tabs using the tail comb, gently pulling the tape "sandwich" apart and remove the extensions from the natural hair. If you encounter any resistance, apply more remover until the bond releases and wait a few more minutes before trying again. It's important to avoid pulling or tugging at the extensions, as this can cause damage to the natural hair.

After the extensions have been removed, you may notice some adhesive residue on the natural hair. Use the soft-bristled brush to gently brush it out. If necessary, you can also apply additional Sajje Hair Collection Tape In Hair Extension Remover to dissolve any remaining adhesive.

Remember to work on one section of the hair at a time, removing one tape in hair extension at a time, and use sectioning clips to hold the hair in place as you work. This will help ensure that you are removing the extensions safely and effectively.

To minimize damage to the natural hair during the removal process, be patient and take your time. Rushing the removal process can cause damage to the natural hair. Additionally, using the right tools such as a tail comb and soft-bristled brush can help minimize damage to the natural hair. It's also important to avoid using heat, as using heat to remove the extensions can cause damage to the natural hair. Stick to the tape removal solution and be patient.

Removing tape in hair extensions may seem intimidating, but with the right tools and techniques, it can be done safely and effectively. By following these step-by-step instructions and tips for minimizing damage to the natural hair, you can remove the tape in hair extensions without causing harm to the hair. Don't forget to properly store the extensions for future use, and always be patient and gentle during the removal process.

Chapter 8

How to Properly Store Tape In Hair Extensions

Properly storing the tape in hair extensions is essential if you plan on reusing them. Here are some steps to follow to ensure that the extensions are well-maintained and ready for future use:

Step 1: Clean the extensions

Before storing the tape in hair extensions, it's important to wash and condition them. This will help to remove any product buildup and keep the extensions soft and silky. Use a clarifying shampoo and a hydrating conditioner, then rinse thoroughly to remove any residue.

Step 2: Dry the extensions

Once you've cleaned the extensions, allow them to air dry completely before storing them. Gently squeeze out any excess water, then lay the extensions flat on a clean towel to dry. Avoid using any heat styling tools, as this can damage the extensions.

Step 3: Remove any excess adhesive

After removing the tape in hair extensions, make sure to remove any excess adhesive from the weft. You can use a 70% alcohol solution or a remover specifically designed for tape in hair extensions to dissolve the adhesive and remove any residue. Replace any tape tabs that may have been damaged during the removal process.

Step 4: Store the extensions

Store the tape in hair extensions in a cool, dry place, away from direct sunlight. Use a hanger or a storage bag specifically designed for hair extensions to prevent tangling and maintain the order of the previous installation. Make sure to label the extensions with their color and length for easy identification if necessary. Another option for storing the tape in hair extensions is to use a hanger. Clip the wefts onto the hanger, making sure they are evenly spaced and not overlapping.

By following these steps, you can store the tape in hair extensions properly and ensure that they are in great condition for future use. Proper maintenance is key to extending the life of the extensions, so take the time to care for them properly

Chapter 9

Re-Installing Tape In Hair Extensions

If you are looking to re-install tape in hair extensions, you'll need to assess their condition before attempting to do so. Consider the length of the extensions, their quality, and the adhesive used to attach them. Assuming they're in good shape, here are the tools you'll need to get started:

1. Tape in hair extensions:
Make sure they're clean and free of any adhesive residue.

2. Double-sided tape:
You'll need fresh double-sided tape to re-install the extensions.

3. Tape remover:
This is optional but can be helpful in removing any adhesive residue from the extensions. We recommend using 70% alcohol.

4. Sectioning clips:
These will be used to section the hair and keep it out of the way while you work.

5. Tail comb:
This will be used to create sections in the hair for the installation.

Once you have everything you need, follow these step-by-step instructions:

1. Wash and condition the hair, making sure to use sulfate-free shampoo and conditioner.

2. Blow-dry the hair completely and use a flat iron to ensure that it is smooth and free of any tangles.

3. Create a horizontal parting about an inch above the nape of the neck and clip the rest of the hair out of the way.

4. Take one of the tape in hair extensions and remove the backing from one side of the tape.

5. Place the extension under the sectioned hair, pressing it firmly against the scalp.

6. Take another extension and remove the backing from one side of the tape.

7. Place the extension directly above the first extension, sandwiching the natural hair between the two tapes.

8. Press the extensions together firmly, ensuring that they are securely attached to the natural hair.

9. Continue adding extensions in a horizontal line, working your way up the head.

10. Once you have installed all of the extensions, use a tail comb to create a parting in the hair about a half-inch above the extensions.

11. Take the top section of the hair and clip it out of the way.

12. Take a small section of hair from underneath the top section and create a parting

13. Remove the backing from one side of the tape on a tape in hair extension and place it under the parting, pressing it firmly against the scalp.

14. Take another extension and remove the backing from one side of the tape.

15. Place the extension directly above the first extension, sandwiching the natural hair between the two tapes.

16. Press the extensions together firmly, ensuring that they are securely attached to the natural hair

Once the tape in hair extensions have been re-installed, you can style the hair as desired. It's important to note that while tape in hair extensions can be re-installed multiple times, it's best to avoid doing so too frequently, as the adhesive on the tapes may become less effective over time, which can result in the extensions falling out or causing damage to the natural hair. If you are using SHC Premium Tape In Hair Extensions by Sajje Hair Collection, keep these tips in mind to ensure successful re-installation, including using a clarifying shampoo before re-installing the extensions, allowing the tapes to rest for at least 24 hours after removal, using 70% alcohol to clean the tapes, and re-taping the extensions after a few uses

Chapter 10

How to Maintain Tape In Hair Extensions

Congratulations on your beautiful new tape in hair extension install! Maintaining them properly is key to keeping them looking great for as long as possible. Here are some tips to help care for the hair and tape in hair extensions after reinstallation:

1. Minimize excessive hair washing:

Washing your hair too often can damage both the natural hair and the tape in hair extensions. Try to limit washing to once or twice a week, and use sulfate free shampoo and conditioner to avoid stripping the hair of natural oils.

2. Use a heat protectant spray:

If you plan to style hair using heat tools, use a heat protectant spray to prevent damage to the hair and the extensions.

3. Avoid chemical treatments:

Chemical treatments, such as coloring or perming, can weaken and damage the tape in hair extensions. If you must dye the hair, avoid getting the dye on the extensions, and consult a professional stylist with experience working with tape in hair extensions.

4. Brush gently:

To prevent tangling and damage to the extensions, use a soft-bristled brush to gently detangle the hair. Start at the bottom of the hair and work your way up, being careful not to tug on the extensions.

5. Use leave-in conditioner:

To keep the hair and extensions moisturized, use a leave-in conditioner. This will help prevent breakage and keep the hair looking healthy.

To maintain and style the tape in hair extensions, we recommend using these products:

1. Sulfate-free shampoo and conditioner:

Using a gentle, sulfate-free formula, such as the L'Oreal Paris EverPure Sulfate-Free Shampoo and Conditioner, is important for preventing damage to the hair and extensions.

2. Heat protectant spray:
We recommend the CHI 44 Iron Guard Thermal Protection Spray to protect the hair from heat damage while styling.

3. Soft-bristled brush:
Use the Wet Brush Original Detangler to gently detangle the hair and prevent damage to the extensions.

4. Leave-in conditioner:
The "It's a 10 Miracle Leave-In Conditioner" or "Knot On My Watch" are both great option to keep the hair and extensions moisturized.

To extend the lifespan of the tape in hair extensions, follow these tips:

1. Sleep with the hair in a bun:
Before going to bed, put the hair in a loose bun to prevent tangling and damage while you sleep.

2. Avoid chlorine and salt water:
Chlorine and salt water can damage the tape in hair extensions, so avoid swimming in pools or the ocean while wearing them.

3. Don't overuse heat tools:
Using heat tools too often can cause damage to both the natural hair and tape in hair extensions. When using heat styling tools, use a heat protectant spray to help minimize damage.

4. Brush regularly:
Brush the hair regularly using a soft-bristle brush to prevent tangling and matting. Start at the ends of the hair and gently work your way up to the roots. Avoid brushing the hair when it's wet, as this can cause breakage.

5. Use sulfate-free products:

Use sulfate-free shampoos and conditioners to prevent the hair from becoming dry and damaged. Sulfates can strip the natural oils from the hair, leaving it brittle and prone to breakage. Look for products that are specifically designed for use with hair extensions.

6. Don't wash the hair too often:

Washing the hair too often can cause the tape in hair extensions to loosen and fall out. Aim to wash the hair no more than two to three times per week.

7. Avoid chlorine and saltwater:

Chlorine and saltwater can cause damage to the hair and tape in hair extensions. If you're going swimming, wear a swim cap or tie the hair up to keep it protected.

8. Get regular maintenance:

It's important to get the tape in hair extensions checked regularly by a professional. They can ensure that the extensions are still securely attached and make any necessary adjustments. It's recommended to have the extensions checked every 4-6 weeks to ensure they are still in good condition.

Additionally, if you notice any signs of damage or tangling, it's important to address these issues as soon as possible to prevent further damage. Don't hesitate to reach out to a professional stylist for guidance on how to care for the extensions properly.

Maintaining tape in hair extensions requires proper care and attention. By following the tips outlined above and using high-quality products, you can help extend the lifespan of the extensions and keep them looking beautiful and healthy. Remember to always be gentle with the hair and seek professional guidance if you have any concerns. With the right care, the tape in hair extensions can give you the stunning, voluminous hair you've always dreamed of.

Chapter 11

Tips and Tricks for Successful Tape In Hair Extension Outcome

As you look to transform your hair look with tape in hair extensions, it's important to note that achieving a natural and seamless outcome requires a lot of attention to detail and careful consideration. With that, before we close, here are a few reminder tips and tricks mentioned on previous pages, for achieving a successful tape in hair extension outcome.

Firstly, avoid installing the extensions too close to the scalp. This can lead to hair breakage and discomfort, so ensure there is a little space between the scalp and the tape in extensions. Secondly, using too many hair extensions can make the hair look bulky and unnatural. A good rule of thumb is to use between 20-40 tape in extension "sandwiches" based on the hair thickness and desired look. Thirdly, ensure you blend the extensions properly with the natural hair to achieve a seamless look. Use a styling tool or hairbrush to blend them effectively. Lastly, not taking care of the extensions properly can reduce their lifespan and cause damage. Be sure to follow the maintenance tips provided in Chapter 10.

Let's now talk about tips for achieving a natural look with tape in hair extensions. Firstly, match the extensions with the natural hair color and texture. This is crucial to achieve a natural look, so select extensions that closely match the natural hair. Secondly, place the extensions strategically to create a seamless look. You can place the extensions in areas where the natural hair is thinner, such as the crown or the sides, ensuring that the tape in is not visible. Thirdly, blending the extensions with the natural hair is essential for a natural look. Use a styling tool or hairbrush to blend them effectively. Lastly, if the extensions are too long, you can cut them to blend with the natural hair. Ensure you cut them in a way that looks natural and seamless.

Want to style the tape in hair extensions creatively? There are numerous ways to enhance the look using tape in hair extensions. You can try the half-up, half-down hairstyle to showcase the fullness that the tape in hair extensions provide. Simply pull the top half of the hair back and secure it with a hair tie or clip. Secondly, braids are a great way to add texture and dimension to the hair. You can create a side braid or a fishtail braid using the tape in hair extensions. Thirdly, the high ponytail is a classic and elegant hairstyle that can be achieved using tape in hair extensions. Gather the hair and the extensions into a high ponytail and secure it with a hair tie. Finally, you can achieve beachy waves using tape in hair extensions by using a curling iron to create loose and natural-looking waves.

To achieve a successful tape in hair extension outcome, it's essential to use high-quality extensions. SHC Premium Tape In Hair Extensions by Sajje Hair Collection are made from 100% Remy human hair and are designed to be long-lasting and easy to maintain. They are available in a range of colors, lengths, and textures to match the natural hair perfectly. Remember, when selecting the length of the tape in hair extensions, it's essential to consider the natural hair length and lifestyle

Chapter 12

Next Steps

Wow, you've just unlocked the secrets to the most flawless and natural-looking hair extensions on the market. Whether you're a stylist, a DIY hair enthusiast, or a hair instructor, we know that you'll appreciate the many benefits of tape in hair extensions.

With our step-by-step guide, you'll learn how to easily install and remove tape in hair extensions without damaging the natural hair. And the best part? Our extensions are made with 100% Remy human hair, ensuring that you'll achieve a seamless blend with the natural hair.

So say goodbye to heavy, uncomfortable extensions that require heat and glue during installation, causing damage to the hair. Our lightweight and easy-to-style tape in hair extensions are long-lasting and can be reused multiple times with proper care. Trust us, you will absolutely love our quality hair products.

At Sajje Hair Collection, we are committed to helping you look and feel your best with our premium tape in hair extensions. Join our community of hair enthusiasts and aspiring professionals by following us on YouTube, Instagram, Facebook, and Twitter. And don't forget to subscribe via email to receive exclusive offers and insider tips from our hair experts.

Ready to take your hair game to the next level? Try our SHC Premium Tape In Hair Extensions today and become part of the Sajje Hair Collection family. We stand behind the quality of our extensions and we know that you'll love them as much as we do. So why wait? Get ready to achieve the hair of your dreams with Sajje Hair Collection

www.ingramcontent.com/pod-product-compliance
Lightning Source LLC
Chambersburg PA
CBHW060258030426
42335CB00014B/1761